The New Mom's Pregnancy Cookbook

A Guide to Nutrition, Recipes, and Meal Plans for a Happy Pregnancy

Virgie W. Miller

COPYRIGHT

TABLE OF CONTENTS

INTRODUCTION

Greetings on your impending birth! You are living through an amazing and thrilling moment in your life, but it is also difficult and stressful. During this time, you can have a lot of questions and worries about how to care for both yourself and your child. Your diet is one of the most crucial components of your overall health. Your health and the growth of your unborn child may be greatly impacted by the foods and beverages you consume. I created this book to empower you to make wise dietary decisions and to provide you access to scrumptious and nourishing recipes that will sustain you and your unborn child during your pregnancy.

The Reasons Behind Writing This Book

I have two children and work as a qualified dietitian. I've always had a strong interest in nutrition and diet, and I wanted to help other expectant women by sharing my expertise. I had a hard time finding trustworthy and useful advice on what to eat and avoid while pregnant with my first kid. Finding meals that were gratifying, simple to make, and appropriate for my evolving requirements and tastes was another challenge for me. Based on my observations and the most recent scientific data, I decided to write my pregnant cookbook. My family, friends, and customers who tried the dishes gave them great feedback, so I kept testing and fine-tuning them until I was satisfied. I'm hoping you'll love them too!

What This Book Has to Offer

The five chapters that make up this book's structure each focus on a distinct phase or facet of your pregnant adventure. Every chapter includes the following:

1. An overview of the typical difficulties and signs of the stage and how diet might help you manage them

2. A section outlining the essential nutrients and dietary categories to concentrate on at that point, along with recommendations for how much and how frequently to eat each.

3. A selection of recipes that employ easy, healthful, and readily available items and

are customized to your preferences and requirements at that point

4. Advice on how to preserve and reheat recipes, as well as how to adjust them to your tastes and the ingredients you have on hand

5. Each dish includes serving sizes and nutritional data so you can monitor your consumption and balance your meals and snacks.

How to Utilize This Book

Rather than serving as a manual or a prescription, this book is meant to be a companion and guide. You are free to use it anyway you see appropriate. The recipes may be followed strictly or modified to your preference. You may follow the recipes in the book exactly every day, or you can substitute recipes from other sources or your own. You have the option to read the book from beginning to end or to go to the chapters or portions that most interest you. The major objective is to promote your health and the development of your unborn child while also enabling you to enjoy food and your pregnancy.

Here are some pointers and recommendations for making the most of the book:

1. Before making any dietary changes, speak with your physician or other health care provider, especially if you have any medical conditions or allergies. Observe the cues your body gives you about hunger and fullness. Aim for balance and variety in your diet by including foods from all the food groups, such as grains, fruits, vegetables, dairy, and healthy fats.

2. Reduce the amount of alcohol, caffeine, and sugar-filled drinks you consume. Consume a lot of water and other liquids.

3. Avoid dangerous or toxic foods such as raw or undercooked meat, seafood, eggs, dairy, unpasteurized milk and cheese, and some fish that are rich in mercury during pregnancy. Instead, practice proper food hygiene and safety.

4. Enjoy yourself periodically, try new meals, tastes, and cultures, and find new ways to appreciate food and your pregnancy. Don't feel bad about giving in to your cravings or favorite foods as long as you do it mindfully and in moderation.

With this book, I wish to empower and encourage you to make the greatest decisions for your child and yourself. I hope your pregnancy is joyous and healthy!

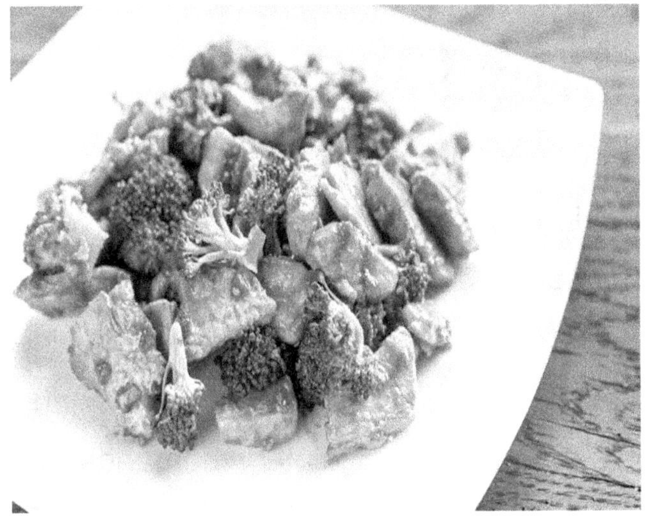

CHAPTER 1

PREGNANCY NUTRITION FUNDAMENTALS

Not only does your body change and develop throughout pregnancy, but so does your unborn child. During this time, you need to provide yourself and your baby with enough energy and nutrients, therefore your dietary demands will vary and rise. Eating a healthy diet may promote your baby's growth and health throughout pregnancy and make you feel good. It can also help you with the physical and mental demands of pregnancy.

Pregnant women's nutritional needs and recommendations

Your pre-pregnancy weight, your exercise level, your age, and the stage of your pregnancy are just a few of the variables that affect how much and what kind of food you require throughout pregnancy. To help you plan your diet and achieve your nutritional demands, there are some basic rules and suggestions.

Calories: To support both your metabolism and the development of your unborn child, you need extra calories throughout pregnancy. But because the additional calories you need are not that great, you don't need to eat for two. The precise number varies based on your unique circumstances, but generally speaking, you could need an additional 300 calories per day during the second trimester and 450 extra calories per day during the third trimester. These additional calories may be obtained from wholesome meals and snacks such as whole grains, nuts, yogurt, cheese, and fruits.

Protein: To grow and repair both your tissues and the tissues of your unborn child, you need extra protein during pregnancy. In addition, protein supports the production of hormones, enzymes, and antibodies by your body—all vital for the health of both you and your unborn child. Pregnant women should consume around 75 grams of protein per day, which is approximately 25 grams more than what is typically advised for women. Animal sources of protein include meat, chicken, fish, eggs, and dairy products. Plant sources of protein include beans, lentils, tofu, nuts, and seeds.

carbs: You and your unborn child both need carbs for energy throughout pregnancy. Additionally, carbs facilitate your body's more effective usage of fat and protein. Pregnant women should have around 175 grams of carbs day, which is approximately the same as what is typically advised for women. Carbohydrates are found in grains, dairy products, fruits, and vegetables. But not every carbohydrate is made equally. Limit simple carbs, which are high in sugar and low in fiber and include sweets, soft drinks, and processed grains. Instead, pick complex carbohydrates, which are rich in fiber and minerals and include whole grains, fruits, and vegetables.

Fat: Throughout pregnancy, fat is necessary for energy production, organ support, and the body's absorption of fat-soluble vitamins including A, D, E, and K. A healthy fat baby's brain and nerve system become stronger. About 65 grams of fat per day is the appropriate amount of fat for pregnant women, which is also the recommended amount for women in general. Oils, butter, margarine, almonds, seeds, avocados, and fatty seafood are all sources of fat. But not all fat is made equally. Saturated or trans fats, like those found in animal fat, coconut oil, palm oil, and hydrogenated oils, should be avoided in favor of unsaturated, healthy fats like those found in olive, canola, sunflower, and fish oils.

Minerals and Vitamins: For both your body's operations and the growth and development of your unborn child, you need vitamins and minerals throughout your pregnancy. The following are a few of the most crucial vitamins and minerals for expectant mothers:

Folate: Your body needs folate, a B vitamin, to build DNA and red blood cells. Neural tube defects are major birth malformations affecting the brain and spine that may be prevented with its assistance. Pregnant women should consume 600 mcg of folate day, which is around double the recommended daily intake for women. Foods like cereals, breads, and pastas that have been fortified with folic acid or naturally occurring foods like leafy green vegetables, beans, lentils, and oranges are good sources of folate. A prenatal vitamin containing 400 micrograms or more of folic acid should be taken daily, beginning before you conceive and continuing until the end of the first trimester.

Iron: Hemoglobin, the protein in your blood that delivers oxygen, is made possible by the mineral iron. To sustain both your growing blood volume and the blood flow to your unborn child, you need extra iron throughout pregnancy. Pregnant women should consume 27 mg of iron per day, which is almost double the recommended daily intake for women. Iron may be obtained from plants such beans, lentils, tofu, spinach, and dried fruits, or from animals like meat, chicken, fish, and eggs. It is recommended that you take a daily prenatal vitamin containing iron, unless your physician instructs you differently.

Calcium: Your body needs calcium to create and maintain healthy bones and teeth. It also promotes healthy blood vessel, muscle, and neuron function. For both your own bone health and the growth of your unborn child's bones, you need calcium throughout pregnancy. Pregnant women should consume 1,000 mg of calcium each day, which is around the same as what is often advised for women. Dairy goods like milk, cheese, and yogurt as well as non-dairy foods like tofu, broccoli, kale, almond milk, orange juice, and fortified soy milk may provide you with calcium. A calcium-containing prenatal vitamin should also be taken daily, unless your doctor instructs you differently.

Vitamin D: A fat-soluble vitamin, vitamin D aids in the body's absorption and use of calcium. Additionally, it supports the healthy operation of both your baby's and your own immune systems. For the sake of both your unborn child's and your own bone health, you must take vitamin D throughout your pregnancy. Pregnant women should take 15 milligrams of vitamin D daily, which is around the same as what is often advised for women. Sunlight exposure, fortified foods (including milk, cereal, and orange juice), and natural sources (such fatty fish, egg yolks, and liver) are the main ways to get vitamin D. It is recommended that you take a daily prenatal vitamin that includes vitamin D, unless your doctor instructs you differently.

Illustrations of Variety and Balance in Meals and Snacks

Here are some examples of balanced and diverse prenatal meals and snacks to help you manage your diet and satisfy your nutritional requirements. The amounts and components may be changed to suit your needs and what's available.

Snack: A cup of yogurt, a handful of mixed nuts and dried fruits, and a glass of orange juice. -

Breakfast: A bowl of whole-grain cereal with low-fat milk and sliced banana, along with a cooked egg.

Lunch: green salad with dressing, a glass of milk, and a turkey and cheese sandwich on whole-wheat bread with lettuce, tomato, and mayonnaise.

Snack: A glass of water and an apple with peanut butter slices

Supper; steamed broccoli, a baked potato with sour cream and chives, baked fish fillet flavored with lemon and herbs, and a glass of water.

Snack: A cup of herbal tea and a piece of whole-wheat bread with jam

Common Myths and Concerns About Nutrition During Pregnancy

You may come across a lot of myths and concerns about nutrition when you are pregnant. While some of them are based on current knowledge or myths, others are based on actual events. These are a few of the most popular ones, along with the real explanation.

Concern: When I'm pregnant, I need to eat for two.

Truth: Since your unborn child is smaller than you, you do not require two meals a day while you are pregnant. Depending on your stage of pregnancy, you only need to eat a little bit more than usual—roughly 300 to 450 extra calories per day. Overeating can result in excessive weight gain, which raises the possibility of complications like preterm delivery, high blood pressure, and gestational diabetes.

Concern: I have to stay away from foods like sushi, cheese, and coffee while I'm pregnant.

Truth is that not all foods should be avoided when pregnant. Foods like raw or undercooked meat, fish, eggs, dairy, unpasteurized milk and cheese, and some fish species that are high in mercury, like king mackerel, shark, and swordfish, should be avoided if they pose a risk to you or your unborn child. As long as the ingredients are cooked or pasteurized and you don't overindulge, you can eat sushi, cheese, and coffee. You may consume up to 6 ounces of cheese daily, 12 ounces of cooked fish per week, and 200 milligrams (approximately one or two cups) of caffeine.

Concern: Taking supplements like vitamins A, C, and E during pregnancy is necessary.

Truth: While pregnant, you should take certain supplements, but not all of them. Unless your doctor instructs you otherwise, you must take a prenatal vitamin daily that contains folic acid, iron, calcium, and vitamin D. It could be difficult to get enough of these nutrients from food alone, but they are vital for both your health and the health of your unborn child. Other supplements, like those containing vitamins A, C, and E, are optional unless prescribed by a physician. Overdosing these vitamins can lead to toxicity or birth defects, which can be dangerous for both you and your unborn child.

Concern: I have to eat a particular diet, like a vegan, vegetarian, or gluten-free one, while I'm pregnant.

The truth is that unless you have a medical condition or allergy that calls for it, you don't need to follow a special diet when you're pregnant.

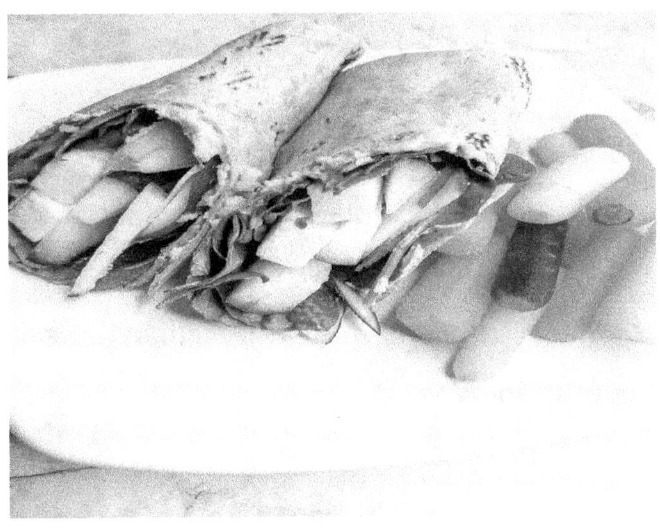

CHAPTER 2

FIRST TRIMESTER RECIPES

Pregnancy's first trimester is a time of wonder and excitement as you learn you are carrying a baby. But, you may also encounter some typical difficulties and symptoms, like nausea, exhaustion, and food aversions, making it a difficult and uncomfortable period. Your baby's health as well as your own may suffer as a result of these problems making it difficult to eat healthily and enjoy your food.

How to Handle Tiredness, Nausea, and Food Aversions

Among the most prevalent and uncomfortable symptoms of the first trimester are fatigue, food aversions, and nausea. They are brought on by the physical adjustments and hormonal shifts your body goes through to support your pregnancy. They can affect your energy levels, digestion, and appetite, even though they are generally harmless. The following are some methods and approaches to deal with these problems and continue eating a healthy diet:

Nausea: Also known as morning sickness, nausea is a feeling of queasiness or vomiting that can strike at any time of the day but is most common in the morning. To mitigate or avoid nausea, consider implementing the following advice:

1. Eat often and in smaller portions rather than in big, heavy ones. Steer clear of foods that are oily, spicy, or strongly scented.
2. Consume cold, bland, or dry foods like ice chips, toast, or crackers.

3. Suck on hard candies, mints, or ginger lozenges - Sip lots of liquids, especially water, ginger ale, or lemonade

4. Put pressure on the inner wrist or wear acupressure wristbands. Inhale clean air and stay away from crowded or smoke-filled areas. Take as much time as you can to relax and rest.

Fatigue: The state of being worn out or exhausted that frequently persists throughout the day is known as fatigue. Try these suggestions to avoid or lessen fatigue:

1. Consume foods rich in nutrients and energy, such as whole grains, yogurt, cheese, nuts, and fruits.

2. Sip hydrating and revitalizing beverages like milk, juice, or water.

3. Steer clear of sweets, soft drinks, and coffee as well as other foods and beverages that are high in sugar and caffeine.

4. Take a daily prenatal vitamin containing folic acid and iron, unless your doctor instructs you otherwise.

5. Get as much rest and sleep as you need, and stick to a regular sleep schedule. - Engage in moderate to regular exercise, like yoga, swimming, or walking. - Seek assistance and support from your partner, family, and friends.

Food Aversions: A food aversion is an uneasiness or revulsion towards a particular food that you would otherwise tolerate or enjoy. They are frequently brought on by the food's flavor, aroma, or appearance. Try these suggestions to avoid or lessen food aversions:

1. Eat mild, simple, or neutral foods like rice, pasta, or potatoes; - Steer clear of foods that make you queasy or repulsed and substitute foods that you can tolerate or enjoy.

2. Consume visually appealing, vibrant, or enjoyable foods like fruit, salad, or pizza. - Try a variety of flavors, textures, and temperatures, such as hot, sour, crunchy, or sweet.

3. Eat foods that bring back memories or are cozy and familiar, like cake, soup, or sandwiches. - Eat a diet that is varied, balanced, and nutrient-dense, incorporating foods from all the food groups.

Recipes for the Initial Three Months

Here are some recipes that are appropriate for this stage of pregnancy to help you manage the difficulties and symptoms of the first trimester while also giving you quick, tasty, and nourishing meals and snacks. They are high in energy, protein, carbs, fat, vitamins, and minerals, and they are made with basic, healthful, and readily available ingredients. They are also made to be aesthetically pleasing, fulfilling, and customizable to your preferences and needs. You can store and reheat the recipes as needed, and you can adjust them to suit your tastes and the available ingredients. At the end of the chapter, you will also find the serving sizes and nutritional information for each recipe.

Smoothie with bananas and peanut butter

This smoothie is a delicious, filling, and healthy way to start the day. It can also help you avoid or lessen fatigue and nausea because it is simple to prepare and digest. It includes peanut butter, which is high in protein and good fat, bananas, which are high in potassium and fiber, and milk, which is high in calcium and vitamin D.

Components

- Two tablespoons of peanut butter
- One large, ripe banana, peeled and sliced
- One cup of nonfat milk
- One-fourth teaspoon vanilla extract
- An optional pinch of cinnamon

Guidelines

- Put all the ingredients in a blender and process them until they are creamy and smooth.
- After pouring into a glass, savor.

Soup with Chicken and Veggies

This soup is warm, calming, and flavorful, making it a satisfying and nourishing meal. It can also help you manage nausea and food aversions because it's simple to prepare and consume. It has vegetables that are high in vitamins and minerals, high-protein and iron chicken, and high-sodium and high-fluid broth.

Components

- Vegetable oil, two tablespoons
- 1 chopped onion
- 2 minced garlic cloves
- 2 peeled and sliced carrots

- 2 sliced celery stalks
- Two cups of water - Four cups of chicken broth
- Two bay leaves
- One teaspoon dried thyme
- Toppings of salt and pepper
- Two cups cooked, chopped or shredded chicken
- 2 tablespoons finely chopped fresh parsley

Guidelines

- Add the oil to a large pot and heat over medium-high heat. Stir in the onion, garlic, carrots, and celery and cook, stirring occasionally, until the vegetables are soft, about 15 minutes.
- Bring to a boil after adding the chicken broth, water, bay leaves, thyme, salt, and pepper. After lowering the heat, cover

and simmer the vegetables for approximately 20 minutes, or until they become tender.

- Cook for an additional ten minutes, or until thoroughly heated, after adding the chicken and parsley.
- Pour the soup into bowls and discard the bay leaves.

Salad with spinach and cheese

This crisp, tangy, and cheesy salad makes a satisfying and healthy snack. You can manage food aversions and cravings with its ease of tossing and customizing. It has cheese, which is high in calcium and protein, dressing, which is high in flavor and healthy fat, and spinach, which is high in iron and folate.

Components

- 1/4 cup of crumbled feta cheese
- 4 cups of baby spinach that have been cleaned and dried
- Two tablespoons of olive oil
- two tablespoons of lemon juice
- two tablespoons of toasted almond slices
- To taste, add salt and pepper.

Guidelines

- Combine the spinach, cheese, and almonds in a big bowl.
- Mix the lemon juice, olive oil, salt, and pepper in a small bowl.
- Pour the salad dressing over it and toss to coat.
- Serve right away or put in the fridge until you're ready to eat.

Avocado and Turkey Sandwich

This sandwich is savory, creamy, and hearty, making it a filling and delicious meal. It can also help you avoid or lessen monotony and boredom because it is simple to assemble and modify. It has bread, which is high in whole grains and carbohydrates, avocado, which is high in fiber and healthy fat, and turkey, which is lean and high in protein.

Components

- Two toasted slices of whole-wheat bread
- Two tablespoons of mayo
- 4 cooked deli turkey slices
- 1/4 peeled and sliced avocado
- 2 dried and cleaned lettuce leaves
- Two dried and cleansed tomato slices
- To taste, add salt and pepper.

Guidelines

- Evenly distribute the mayonnaise across the slices of bread.
- Arrange one slice of bread with the turkey, avocado, lettuce, and tomato on top.
- To taste, add salt and pepper to the dish before serving.
- Place the remaining piece of bread on top and cut it in half.
- Savor it with some milk or water in a glass.

Berries and Oatmeal

This soft, sweet, and filling oatmeal makes for a warm and comforting breakfast. It can also help you manage nausea and food aversions because it is simple to prepare and alter. It has berries, which are high in antioxidants and vitamin C, oatmeal, which is high in fiber and complex carbohydrates, and milk, which is high in calcium and protein.

Components

- 1/4 cup of frozen or fresh berries, such as strawberries, raspberries, or blueberries
- 1/2 cup of rolled oats
- 1 cup of water
- a dash of salt;
- One-fourth cup of skim milk
- One tablespoon of maple syrup or honey
- An optional dash of nutmeg or cinnamon

Guidelines

- Heat a small saucepan with the oats, water, and salt over medium-high heat. Once the oats are soft and creamy, reduce the heat and simmer for approximately 10 minutes, stirring from time to time.

- Once the berries are soft and juicy, stir them in and cook for an additional five minutes.
- Spoon the oatmeal into a bowl, then pour in the milk and maple syrup or honey.
- If preferred, add a dash of nutmeg or cinnamon and savor.

Hummus with Vegetable Wraps

With its crunchy, creamy, and zesty texture, this wrap makes a light and refreshing lunch. Additionally, it is simple to assemble and move, which can lessen or avoid boredom and exhaustion. It includes veggies, which are high in vitamins and minerals, whole grains and carbohydrates, and hummus, which is high in protein and healthy fat.

Components

- One whole-wheat tortilla,
- two tablespoons of hummus,
- one tablespoon each of crumbled feta cheese and grated carrot,
- one-fourth cup each of shredded lettuce and sliced cucumber,
- one tablespoon each of lemon juice
- To taste, add salt and pepper.

Guidelines

- Place the tortilla on a level surface and cover it evenly with hummus.
- Over the hummus, scatter the cheese, carrot, cucumber, and lettuce.
- Sprinkle salt and pepper on top of the filling and drizzle with lemon juice.
- Roll the tortilla tightly after folding the sides over the center and the bottom edge over the filling.

- Enjoy with a glass of juice or water after cutting in half.

Cheese and Apple Muffins

These muffins are fluffy, cheesy, and moist—a delightful combination of sweet and savory flavors. Additionally, they are simple to store and bake, which can help you avoid or lessen boredom and hunger. They include cheese, which is high in calcium and protein, apples, which are high in fiber and vitamin C, and flour, which is high in whole grains and carbohydrates.

Components

- Two cups of flour that's whole-wheat
- Two teaspoons of baking powder
- One-half teaspoon baking soda
- One-fourth teaspoon each of salt and nutmeg

- 1/4 cup softened butter
- One-fourth cup of brown sugar
- Two eggs
- One cup of nonfat milk
- One cup of grated cheddar cheese
- One teaspoon of vanilla extract
- One cup of diced and peeled apple

Guidelines

- Set aside a 12-cup muffin tin and line it with paper liners. Preheat the oven to 375°F.
- Mix the flour, baking soda, baking powder, salt, and nutmeg in a big bowl.
- Using an electric mixer, beat the butter and sugar in a separate bowl until the mixture is light and fluffy. Add the eggs one at a time, beating well after each addition. Add the vanilla and milk, and stir.

- Mixing until just combined, add the wet ingredients to the dry ingredients. Mix in the apple and cheese.
- About three-quarters of the way full, spoon the batter into the muffin cups that have been prepared.
- When a toothpick inserted in the center comes out clean, bake for 18 to 20 minutes.
- After allowing the muffins to cool somewhat in the pan, move them to a wire rack to finish cooling.
- Savor it with some juice or milk in a glass.

Pasta with Sauced Tomatoes

Tender, saucy, and flavorful, this pasta makes a perfect, cozy supper. It can also help you manage nausea and food aversions because it is simple to cook and modify. It has cheese, which is high in calcium and protein, tomato sauce, which is high in lycopene and vitamin A, and pasta, which is high in complex and simple carbohydrates.

Components

- 8 ounces of whole-wheat pasta, like fusilli, penne, or spaghetti
- 2 tablespoons of olive oil
- 1 chopped onion - 2 minced garlic cloves
- A single, 28-oz can of crushed tomatoes
- One teaspoon dried oregano
- Two teaspoons dried basil
- Taste and adjust salt and pepper.
- Grate 1/4 cup of parmesan cheese.

Guidelines

- As directed on the package, cook the pasta until it's al dente. Empty and put back into the pot.

- The oil should be heated to medium-high heat in a big skillet. Add the onion and garlic, and cook for about 10 minutes, or until soft and golden, stirring now and then.

- Bring to a boil after adding the tomatoes, basil, oregano, salt, and pepper. After lowering the heat, simmer the sauce, uncovered, for approximately fifteen minutes, or until it thickens and bubbles.

- -After spooning the sauce over the pasta, top with cheese.

- Savor it with a bread slice or a green salad.

Smoothie for Morning Sickness Soother

Components:

- 1 ripe banana
- One-half cup Greek yogurt, plain
- Half a cup of frozen strawberries and ha
- a cup of frozen mango chunks.
- One tablespoon honey, if desired
- Half a cup of almond milk or coconut water

Guidelines

- After peeling, chop the banana into large pieces.
- Put the frozen mango chunks, frozen strawberries, Greek yogurt, banana chunks, honey (if using), and almond milk or coconut water in a blender.
- Blend until creamy and smooth.

- Transfer into a glass and consume as a cool breakfast or snack to lessen symptoms of morning sickness.

Stir-fried Ginger-Lime Chicken

Ingredients:

- 1 pound thinly sliced boneless, skinless chicken breast;
- 2 minced garlic cloves;
- 1 tablespoon olive oil
- One tablespoon of freshly grated ginger
- One thinly sliced red bell pepper
- One cup of snap peas
- One lime, zest, and juice
- Two tablespoons of low-sodium soy sauce
- One tablespoon of honey and cooked brown rice ready to be served

Guidelines

- In a large skillet or wok, heat the olive oil over medium-high heat.

- Add the sliced chicken breast to the skillet and cook for 5 to 6 minutes, or until browned and cooked through.

- Cook the grated ginger and minced garlic in the skillet for a further one to two minutes, or until fragrant.

- Add the snap peas and sliced red bell pepper, and cook for 3–4 minutes, or until the veggies are crisp-tender.

- Combine the lime zest, lime juice, soy sauce, and honey in a small bowl. Toss to coat the chicken and vegetables in the skillet after pouring the mixture over them.

- Simmer for a further one to two minutes, or until the sauce somewhat thickens.

- Transfer the stir-fried ginger-lime chicken to cooked brown rice and savor!

Rich Avocado and Chickpea Salad

Ingredients:

- One ripe avocado, chopped
- One fifteen-ounce can of rinsed and drained chickpeas
- 1/4 cup diced red onion;
- 1/4 cup chopped fresh cilantro;
- 1 lemon's juice
- To serve, combine 2 tablespoons extra-virgin olive oil, baby spinach, or mixed greens, salt, and pepper to taste.

Guidelines:

- Combine the diced red onion, chopped cilantro, chickpeas, and avocado in a big mixing bowl.
- Pour extra virgin olive oil and lemon juice over the salad ingredients.
- Toss gently to ensure that everything is evenly coated after adding salt and pepper to taste.
- Top baby spinach or mixed greens with the creamy avocado and chickpea salad.
- Savor is a nutritious and light lunch or dinner option that is perfect for the first trimester of pregnancy.

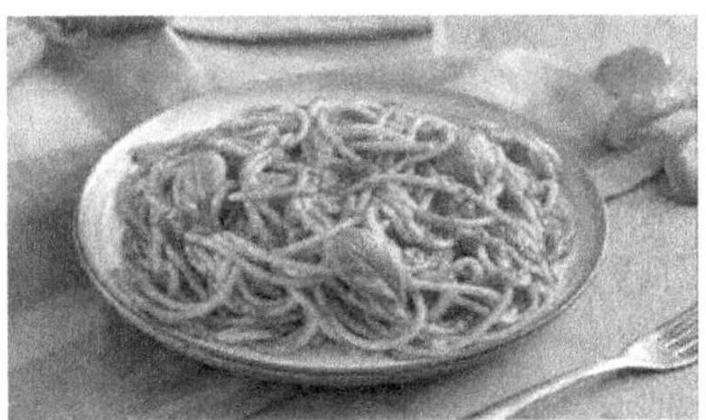

CHAPTER 3

SECOND TRIMESTER RECIPES

Pregnancy is a joyful and relieving time during the second trimester when you can feel your growing baby. It's also a time of greater demand and accountability because you have to feed your baby enough calories and protein to support both your health and their development. In addition to supporting your baby's growth and health, eating well during the second trimester can help you feel upbeat, content, and confident.

Why You Require More Protein and Calories in the Second Trimester

Your baby develops quickly in the second trimester and hits significant developmental milestones like the formation of muscles, organs, and bones. You require more protein and calories than you did previously to support this growth. The energy that your body and your baby use for different tasks and activities is measured in calories. The building block of both your body and your unborn child's, protein aids in the formation and maintenance of tissues, hormones, enzymes, and antibodies.

Several factors, including your age, activity level, pre-pregnancy weight, and pregnancy stage, determine how many calories and protein you need during the second trimester. To help you plan your diet and meet your needs, there are some general guidelines and recommendations.

Calories: During the second trimester, you require approximately 340 extra calories per day or about 40 more than during the first trimester. These additional calories can be obtained from wholesome meals and snacks like whole grains, nuts, yogurt, cheese, and fruits. Sweets, soft drinks, and fast food are examples of foods and beverages that are high in calories, fat, and sugar but low in nutrients. These can cause excessive weight gain, which raises the risk of complications like gestational diabetes, high blood pressure, and preterm delivery.

Protein: In the second trimester, you require approximately 71 grams of protein daily, which is approximately 21 grams more than in the first. Meat, poultry, fish, eggs, and dairy products are examples of animal-based protein sources. Plant sources of protein include beans, lentils, tofu, nuts, and seeds. Aim for balance and diversity in your protein intake, getting it from both plant and animal sources.

Appetizers for the Recess Phase

Here are some recipes that are appropriate for the second trimester that will help you meet your calorie and protein needs while also giving you tasty, filling meals and snacks that are high in protein. They are high in energy, protein, carbs, fat, vitamins, and minerals, and they are made with basic, healthful, and readily available ingredients. They are also made to be aesthetically pleasing, fulfilling, and customizable to your preferences and needs. You can store and reheat the recipes as needed, and you can adjust them to suit your tastes and the available ingredients. At the end of the chapter, you will also find the serving sizes and nutritional information for each recipe.

Casserole with Beef and Vegetables

With its tender, saucy, and cheesy texture, this casserole makes a satisfying and tasty supper. Additionally, it is simple to prepare and freeze, which can lessen or avoid boredom and exhaustion. It has vegetables that are high in vitamins and minerals, high-protein and high in calcium cheese, and beef that is high in iron and protein.

Components

- A single tablespoon of olive oil
- One pound of lean ground beef
- one chopped onion; two minced garlic cloves
- One 10.5-oz can of mushroom cream soup
- One-fourth cup of water

- One teaspoon of sauce from Worcestershire.
- Two cups of thawed frozen mixed vegetables
- Salt and pepper to taste
- Four cups of cooked mashed potatoes - Two cups of shredded cheddar cheese

Guidelines

- Grease a 9x13-inch baking dish with cooking spray and preheat the oven to 375°F.
- Heat the oil in a big skillet over medium-high heat. When the beef is browned and the onion is soft, add the beef, onion, and garlic. Cook, breaking up the meat with a spatula, for about 15 minutes. Eliminate the surplus fat.
- Bring to a boil after adding the soup, Worcestershire sauce, water, salt, and

pepper. Lower the temperature and let it gently simmer for approximately ten minutes, stirring from time to time, until the sauce thickens.

- Evenly spoon the beef mixture into the baking dish that has been preheated. Evenly distribute the vegetables over the beef mixture by scattering them on top. Evenly distribute the cheese over the vegetables after sprinkling them on. Evenly distribute the mashed potatoes with a spoon over the cheese.
- Bake for 25 to 30 minutes, until the cheese has melted and the potatoes are golden.
- Savor with a bread slice or a green salad.

Stir-fried Broccoli and Chicken

This savory, crunchy, and spicy stir-fry makes a quick and simple dinner. It is also simple to cook and adapt, so you can experiment with different flavors and cuisines and add more diversity and variety to your diet. It includes rice, which is high in complex carbohydrates and carbohydrates overall, broccoli, which is high in vitamin C and folate, and chicken, which is lean and full of protein.

Components

- Soy sauce, two tablespoons
- 1/4 teaspoon of red pepper flakes
- 1 tablespoon of cornstarch
- One pound of thinly sliced, skinless, boneless chicken breasts
- Two tablespoons of vegetable oil
- Four cups of florets of broccoli
- Two minced garlic cloves
- Two tsp toasted sesame seeds
- Four cups cooked brown rice

Guidelines

- Combine the red pepper flakes, cornstarch, and soy sauce in a small bowl. Toss to coat after adding the chicken.Refrigerate for a duration of fifteen minutes.

- Heat the oil in a large skillet or wok over high heat.

- Stir-fry the chicken for ten minutes or until it turns golden and is thoroughly cooked. Move to a platter and maintain the heat.

- In the same skillet or wok, add the broccoli and garlic and stir-fry until crisp-tender, about 5 minutes.

- Add the chicken back to the skillet or wok and mix everything. Add the sesame seeds and stir.

- Enjoy with a side of rice.

Pasta with Sauced Tomatoes

Tender, saucy, and flavorful, this pasta makes a perfect, cozy supper. It can also help you manage nausea and food aversions because it is simple to cook and modify. It has cheese, which is high in calcium and protein, tomato sauce, which is high in lycopene and vitamin A, and pasta, which is high in complex and simple carbohydrates.

Components

- 8 ounces of whole-wheat pasta, like fusilli, penne, or spaghetti
- 2 tablespoons of olive oil
- 1 chopped onion
- 2 minced garlic cloves
- A single, 28-oz can of crushed tomatoes
- One teaspoon dried oregano

- Two teaspoons dried basil
- Taste and adjust salt and pepper.
- Grate 1/4 cup of parmesan cheese.

Guidelines

- As directed on the package, cook the pasta until it's al dente. Pour back into the pot after emptying.
- Heat the oil in a big skillet over medium-high heat. Add the onion and garlic, and cook for about 10 minutes, or until soft and golden, stirring now and then.
- Bring to a boil after adding the tomatoes, basil, oregano, salt, and pepper. Once the sauce has thickened, reduce the heat and simmer, uncovered, for approximately 15 minutes.
- After spooning the sauce over the pasta, top with cheese.

- Savor it with a bread slice or a green salad.

Cheese and Vegetable Quesadillas

These crunchy, cheesy, and veggie-packed quesadillas make a simple and quick snack. Additionally, they are simple to prepare and adapt, so you can experiment with different flavors and cuisines and increase the diversity and variety of your diet. They contain cheese, which is high in calcium and protein, vegetables, which are high in vitamins and minerals, and tortillas, which are high in whole grains and carbohydrates.

Components

- Four whole-wheat tortillas
- one cup of shredded cheddar cheese
- one-fourth cup of rinsed and drained black beans;

- one-fourth cup of thawed corn kernels
- one-fourth cup of diced red bell pepper
- two tablespoons of chopped cilantro
- one-fourth teaspoon of cumin; salt and pepper to taste
- two teaspoons of vegetable oil
- Serve with salsa, guacamole, and sour cream (if desired).

Guidelines

- Combine the cheese, beans, corn, cilantro, cumin, bell pepper, and salt and pepper in a small bowl.
- On a level surface, place two tortillas and equally distribute the cheese mixture up over them. Place the remaining tortillas on top and gently press to seal.
- In a large skillet, heat the oil over medium-high heat. One quesadilla should be carefully transferred to the

skillet and cooked for about three minutes on each side, or until crisp and golden. Continue making the other quesadilla.

- Cut into wedges and, if preferred, serve with guacamole, salsa, and sour cream.

Pizza with cheese and tomatoes

With its crispy, cheesy, and tomatoey flavor, this pizza makes a tasty and simple snack. It is also simple to prepare and alter, allowing you to experiment with different flavors and cuisines and diversify your diet. It has cheese, which is high in calcium and protein, tomato sauce, which is high in lycopene and vitamin A, and pizza crust, which is high in whole grains and carbohydrates.

Components
- 1/2 cup pizza sauce

- 1 12-inch whole-wheat pizza crust
- One cup of mozzarella cheese, shredded

Grated parmesan cheese, 1/4 cup

2 tablespoons chopped fresh basil

Guidelines

- Spread the pizza crust out on a baking sheet and preheat the oven to 375°F.
- Evenly cover the pizza crust with the pizza sauce, leaving a 1/2-inch border all the way around.
- Evenly distribute the mozzarella and parmesan cheeses on top of the pizza sauce.
- Bake the cheese for 15 to 20 minutes, or until it is bubbly and melted.
- After sprinkling the pizza with basil, cut it into slices.
- Savor it with a glass of milk or a green salad.

Bean and Veggie Chili

This spicy, hearty, and bean-packed chili makes for a warm and comforting supper. It can also help you avoid or lessen boredom and fatigue because it is simple to cook and freeze. It has vegetables that are rich in vitamins and minerals, beans that are high in protein and fiber, and spices that are high in flavor and antioxidants.

Components
- Two tablespoons of vegetable oil
- one chopped onion; two minced garlic cloves
- one chopped green bell pepper; and one chopped red bell pepper
- Two diced carrots (peeled)
- Two diced celery stalks

- Two fifteen-ounce cans of rinsed and drained black beans;
- Two fifteen-ounce cans of rinsed and drained kidney beans
- Two 14.5-oz cans of diced tomatoes and juice
- Two cups of vegetable broth
- One tablespoon each of cumin, chili powder, and oregano
- Season with salt and pepper
- Garnish with chopped green onions, sour cream, and shredded cheddar cheese (optional)

Guidelines

- Heat the oil in a large pot over medium-high heat. Cook the onion, garlic, bell peppers, carrots, and celery for approximately 20 minutes, stirring periodically, or until they become soft and tender.

- Bring the mixture to a boil after adding the beans, tomatoes, broth, cumin, oregano, chili powder, and salt and pepper. Once the chili is thick and bubbly, reduce the heat and simmer, uncovered, for approximately half an hour.
- Spoon the chili into individual bowls and garnish with sour cream, cheese, and green onions, if preferred.
- Savor it with a glass of water or a piece of bread.

Stuffed bell peppers with Quinoa

Components:

- 4 large bell peppers, cut off the tops and seeds;
- 1 cup rinsed quinoa

- Two cups water or vegetable broth
- One tablespoon of olive oil
- One chopped onion
- Two minced garlic cloves
- One chopped zucchini
- One cup of halved cherry tomatoes
- One cup of cooked black beans,
- one teaspoon of ground cumin, and one teaspoon of paprika
- To taste, add salt and pepper
- If desired, add 1/2 cup of shredded cheese

Guidelines

- Set the oven's temperature to 375°F or 190°C.
- Place the quinoa and water or vegetable broth in a medium saucepan. After bringing it to a boil, lower the heat to a simmer, cover, and cook the quinoa for

about fifteen minutes, or until it is fluffy and cooked.

- Heat the olive oil in a big skillet over medium heat. Cook for approximately five minutes, or until the diced onion is soft.

- Fill the skillet with the diced zucchini, chopped cherry tomatoes, and minced garlic. Simmer the vegetables for an additional five minutes, or until they are soft.

- Add the black beans, ground cumin, paprika, cooked quinoa, salt, and pepper. To allow the flavors to meld, simmer for an additional two to three minutes.

- Gently press the quinoa and vegetable mixture into the bell peppers, making sure to pack them in tightly.

- If you're using cheese, then top the stuffed bell peppers with it.

- Transfer the stuffed bell peppers to a baking dish and tent them with foil. Bake for 25 to 30 minutes, or until the peppers are soft, in an oven that has been preheated.
- If desired, top the hot bell peppers with quinoa and fresh herbs.

Foil packets with asparagus and salmon

Components:

- One pound of trimmed asparagus spears
- Four salmon filets
- Two tablespoons of olive oil
- Two minced garlic cloves
- One thinly sliced lemon
- Season with salt and pepper
- Garnish with fresh dill (optional)

Guidelines:

- Set the oven's temperature to 400°F, or 200°C.

- Cut four big pieces of foil that are big enough to encircle a salmon filet and a couple of asparagus spears.

- In the middle of each foil piece, place a salmon fillet.

- Surround each salmon fillet with a few spears of asparagus.

- Combine the minced garlic and olive oil in a small bowl. Pour the mixture over the asparagus and salmon.

- Top each salmon filet with two slices of lemon.

- Add salt and pepper to taste and season everything.

- To make sealed packets, fold the foil over the salmon and asparagus.

- Transfer the foil packets to a baking sheet and bake for 15 to 20 minutes, or until the asparagus is soft and the salmon is cooked through.
- Open the foil packets carefully, watching out for steam.
- If desired, top the salmon and asparagus with freshly chopped dill and serve hot.

Quinoa Salad with Mango and Black Beans

Ingredients:

- 1 cup rinsed quinoa, 2 cups water,
- 1 diced ripe mango,
- 1 diced red bell pepper,
- 1/2 cup cooked black beans,
- 1/4 cup chopped fresh cilantro
- One lime juice;
- Two tablespoons extra virgin olive oil;
- Season with salt and pepper
- Serve with baby spinach or mixed greens

Guidelines

- Put the quinoa and water in a medium-sized saucepan. After bringing it to a boil, lower the heat to a simmer, cover, and cook the quinoa for about fifteen minutes, or until it is fluffy and cooked.

- Place the cooked quinoa, diced mango, diced red bell pepper, cooked black beans, and fresh cilantro in a large mixing bowl.

- Combine the extra-virgin olive oil and lime juice in a small bowl. Toss the quinoa salad to ensure that everything is evenly coated after adding the dressing.

- To taste, add salt and pepper to the salad.

- Present the quinoa salad with mango and black beans on a bed of baby spinach or mixed greens.
- Savor it as a light and revitalizing meal that is rich in vitamins, fiber, and protein—all of which are crucial for the second trimester of pregnancy.

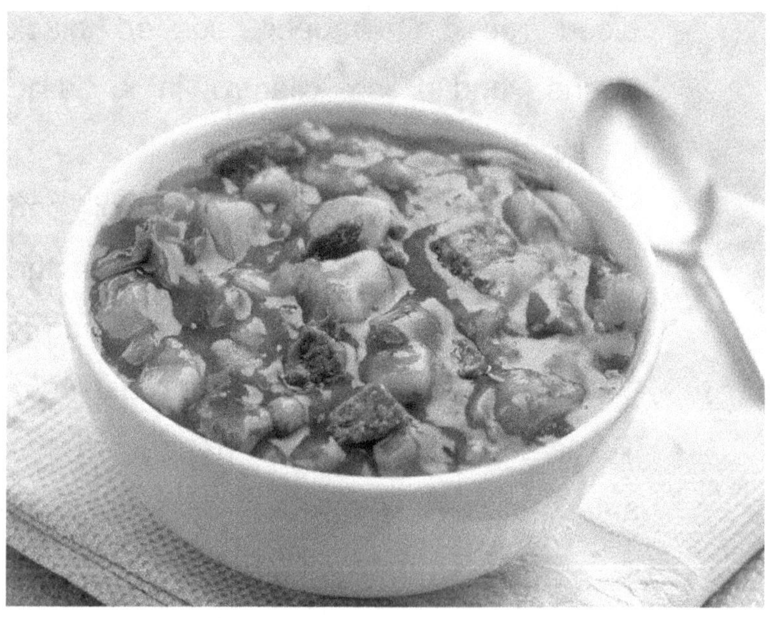

CHAPTER 4

THIRD TRIMESTER RECIPES

When you approach the third trimester of pregnancy, you should be feeling excited and ready to meet your little one. But it's also a difficult and uncomfortable time, with common problems and symptoms like heartburn, constipation, swelling, and nesting. Your baby's health as well as your own may suffer as a result of these problems making it difficult to eat healthily and enjoy your food.

How to Handle Constipation, Swelling, Nesting, and Heartburn

Several of the most prevalent and uncomfortable third-trimester symptoms include heartburn, constipation, swelling, and nesting. They are brought on by the physical strain and hormonal adjustments your body makes to accommodate your developing child. They can affect your comfort, digestion, and appetite, even though they are generally harmless. The following are some methods and approaches to deal with these problems and continue eating a healthy diet:

Heartburn: This burning feeling in your throat or chest is commonly experienced after eating or after lying down. The reason behind it is that your lower esophageal sphincter relaxes and your baby puts pressure on your esophagus, causing acid from your stomach to reflux into it. To mitigate or avoid heartburn, consider implementing the following advice:

1. Eat frequent, small meals instead of large, heavy ones. Steer clear of foods that are fatty, acidic, or spicy, like

tomatoes, citrus fruits, chocolate, and fried foods.

2. Drink fluids instead of carbonated, caffeinated, or alcoholic drinks in between meals.

3. To increase salivation and balance acid after meals, chew gum or suck on hard candies, mints, or lozenges.

4. Use pillows or wedges to raise your head and upper body when you're lying down to stop acid reflux.

5. Take antacids or other prescription drugs as directed by your doctor to relieve the symptoms.

Constipation: Constipation is defined as the inability or difficulty to pass stool, which can lead to discomfort, cramping, and bloating. The pressure of your baby compressing your colon and your elevated progesterone levels slowing down your intestinal motility are the causes. Try these suggestions to avoid or lessen constipation:

1. Consume a diet rich in fiber-containing foods, such as fruits, vegetables, whole grains, beans, and nuts. - Stay hydrated by drinking lots of water to soften your stools and avoid dehydration.

2. To improve blood circulation and stimulate bowel movements, engage in regular, moderate exercise such as yoga, swimming, or walking. - Steer clear of high-sugar, low-fiber foods like white bread, pastries, and candy, as they can exacerbate constipation. To facilitate the passage of feces, take laxatives or stool softeners as directed by your physician.

Swelling: Swelling is the build-up of fluid in your tissues and can cause your face, hands, feet, and ankles to feel swollen, tight, and uncomfortable. It results from the pressure of your baby and the relaxation of your blood vessels, which in turn causes an increase in blood volume and a decrease in blood flow in your veins. Try these suggestions to avoid or lessen swelling:

1. Consume foods low in sodium, like fresh produce, lean meats, and processed foods; foods high in sodium, like canned goods, processed foods, and salty snacks, can cause fluid retention.

2. Consume hydrating and diuretic liquids, like water, juice, or herbal tea; stay away from dehydrating or stimulant liquids, like soda, coffee, or alcohol, as these can exacerbate swelling.

3. Use pillows or stools to raise your legs and feet when seated or lying down to increase blood flow and decrease fluid retention.

4. Wear loose-fitting, comfy clothes and shoes; steer clear of constrictive jewelry like bracelets, rings, and socks, which can worsen swelling and reduce blood flow. To ease the pressure and pain, gently massage your hands and feet, or have a partner, family member, or friend do it for you.

Nesting: Nesting is the instinctive desire to prepare your home—especially the room where your baby will be born—by organizing, cleaning, and decorating it. Hormonal changes and the emotional excitement that comes with getting closer to your due date are the causes. Nesting can be productive and enjoyable, but it can also be draining and stressful, particularly if you overdo it or disregard your personal needs. You can attempt the following advice to stop or lessen the negative effects of nesting:

1. Make a list of everything you need to do and everything you want to do, prioritize your tasks, and start with the most important things. - Ask your partner, family, and friends for support and assistance. Give them some of the housework or errands to run. - Consider using a professional service if you have the funds.

2. Make sure you don't push yourself past your comfort zone or disregard your body's signals. Instead, take regular breaks and rest as needed.

3. Consume quick and easy meals like fruits, nuts, yogurt, cheese, and whole

grains; stay away from time-consuming and unhealthy meals like fast food, junk food, and complicated dishes that can deplete your energy and resources.

4. As long as you and your child are safe and comfortable, don't worry about perfection or details. Instead, enjoy the process and the result and recognize your efforts and accomplishments.

Recipes for the Third Stage of Pregnancy

These recipes are appropriate for the third trimester of pregnancy and will help you manage the difficulties and symptoms while also giving you some easy, soothing, and hydrating meals and snacks. They are high in fiber, liquid, calcium, and vitamin C, and they are prepared with basic, healthful, and readily available ingredients. Additionally, they are made to be calming, enticing, and customizable to your preferences and needs. You can store and reheat the recipes as needed, and you can adjust them to suit your tastes and the available ingredients. At the end of the chapter, you will also find the serving sizes and nutritional information for each recipe.

Berries and Oatmeal

This soft, sweet, and filling oatmeal makes for a warm and comforting breakfast. It can also help you manage nausea and food aversions because it is simple to prepare and alter. It has berries, which are high in antioxidants and vitamin C, oatmeal, which is high in fiber and complex carbohydrates, and milk, which is high in calcium and protein.

Components

- 1/4 cup of frozen or fresh berries, such as strawberries, raspberries, or blueberries;
- 1/2 cup of rolled oats;
- 1 cup of water; a dash of salt;
- One-fourth cup of skim milk
- One tablespoon of maple syrup or honey
- An optional dash of nutmeg or cinnamon

Guidelines

- Heat a small saucepan with the oats, water, and salt over medium-high heat. Once the oats are soft and creamy, reduce the heat and simmer for approximately 10 minutes, stirring from time to time.
- Once the berries are soft and juicy, stir them in and cook for an additional five minutes.

- Spoon the oatmeal into a bowl, then pour in the milk and maple syrup or honey.
- If preferred, add a dash of nutmeg or cinnamon and savor.

A parfait of yogurt and granola

This fruity, crunchy, and smooth parfait makes for a refreshing, creamy snack. It is also simple to make and adapt, so you can experiment with different flavors and cuisines and add more diversity and variety to your diet. It has granola, which is high in fiber and complex carbohydrates, fruit, which is high in antioxidants and vitamin C, and yogurt, which is high in calcium and protein.

Components

- One cup of vanilla or plain low-fat yogurt
- 1/4 cup of homemade or store-bought granola

- One-fourth cup of frozen or fresh fruit, like mangoes, peaches, or berries
- One tablespoon (optional) of maple syrup or honey

Guidelines

- Arrange half of the fruit, half of the granola, and half of the yogurt in a small bowl.
- Continue with the leftover fruit, granola, and yogurt.
- Enjoy with a drizzle of honey or maple syrup, if preferred.

Tea with Fruit and Herbs

This aromatic, sweet, and refreshing tea makes a warm, comforting beverage. You can manage nausea and food aversions with its ease of brewing and customization. It has fruit, which is rich in vitamin C and antioxidants, and herbal tea, which is flavorful and high in fluid content.

Components

- Two glasses of water
- Two bags of herbal tea, like ginger, mint, or chamomile
- One-fourth cup of frozen or fresh fruit, like apples, lemons, or oranges
- One tablespoon of sugar or honey, if desired

Guidelines

- Bring a small saucepan of water to a boil over high heat.
- .Take off the heat and stir in the fruit and tea bags. Once the fruit is soft and the tea has been infused, cover and steep for approximately ten minutes.

- After straining the tea into a large mug, throw away the fruit and the tea bags. Enjoy after adding the sugar or honey, if preferred.

Meatballs with vegetables and turkey soup

Ingredients:

- One pound of lean ground turkey
- half a cup of breadcrumbs
- One egg - Two minced garlic cloves
- A quarter of a cup of grated Parmesan cheese
- one teaspoon of dry oregano
- Two tablespoons of olive oil
- 1/2 teaspoon dried basil
- Salt and pepper to taste
- One diced onion;
- Two diced carrots;
- Two diced celery stalks
- 2 cups baby spinach

- 6 cups low-sodium chicken broth
- Cooked pasta, optional

Guidelines

- Combine the ground turkey, breadcrumbs, egg, minced garlic, grated Parmesan cheese, dried basil, dried oregano, salt, and pepper in a sizable mixing bowl. Blend until thoroughly blended.
- Using the turkey mixture, form tiny meatballs with a diameter of roughly one inch.
- In a big pot over medium heat, warm the olive oil. Cook the diced onion, carrots, and celery for approximately five minutes, or until they become tender.
- Fill the pot with the chicken broth and simmer.

- Once the broth is simmering, carefully place the meatballs in it and cook for 8 to 10 minutes, or until they are thoroughly cooked.
- Add the baby spinach and cook, stirring, for a further one to two minutes, or until wilted.
- Just before serving, if desired, mix cooked pasta into the soup.
- If desired, top the hot turkey and vegetable meatball soup with fresh herbs.

Roasted vegetables and salmon with honey mustard on a sheet pan

Ingredients

- 1 pound halved baby potatoes;
- 2 tablespoons whole grain mustard;
- 2 tablespoons honey;
- 1 tablespoon olive oil;

- 4 salmon fillets;
- Two cups of cauliflower florets;
- Two cups of broccoli florets
- Season with salt and pepper
- Present with lemon wedges

Guidelines

- Set the oven's temperature to 400°F, or 200°C. Put parchment paper on the bottom of a large baking sheet.
- To make the honey mustard glaze, combine the olive oil, honey, and whole-grain mustard in a small bowl.
- Arrange the salmon filets on half of the baking sheet that has been ready.
- On the opposite side of the baking sheet, arrange the baby potatoes, broccoli florets, and cauliflower florets.

- Pour the honey mustard glaze over the veggies and salmon filets, tossing to ensure that everything is evenly coated.
- Add salt and pepper to taste and season everything.
- Roast for 15 to 20 minutes, or until the vegetables are soft and the salmon is cooked through, in a preheated oven.
- Present the heated honey mustard salmon along with the roasted vegetables, providing lemon wedges for squeezing over the salmon.

Chicken Breast Stuffed with Feta and Spinach

Ingredients

- Four skinless, boneless chicken breast.
- 2 cups of fresh spinach leaves
- 1/2 cup of feta cheese crumbles
- 2 minced garlic cloves

- One tablespoon olive oil

- Toppings of salt and pepper

- Toothpicks

Guidelines

- Turn the oven on to 375°F, or 190°C. Grease a baking dish with cooking spray.

- Over medium heat, preheat the olive oil in a skillet. Add the minced garlic and cook until fragrant, about 1 minute.

- Add the fresh spinach to the skillet and cook for two to three minutes, or until wilted.

- Take the skillet off of the burner and mix in the feta cheese crumbles until well combined.

- Gently cut a pocket into each chicken breast with a sharp knife.

- Stuff the spinach and feta mixture into each pocket of a chicken breast.

- Use toothpicks to fasten the pockets shut.
- Add salt and pepper to taste when spicing the stuffed chicken breasts.
- Transfer the stuffed chicken breasts to the ready baking dish.
- Bake for 25 to 30 minutes, or until the chicken is thoroughly cooked, in an oven that has been preheated.
- Give the chicken a few minutes to rest before taking out the toothpicks.
- Present the heated Chicken Breast with Stuffed Spinach and Feta along with your preferred sides.

Savor this tasty and nourishing dish while you're pregnant in the third trimester!

Some Advice on How to Prepare Your Freezer and Pantry for Postpartum

As your due date draws near, you might want to fill your freezer and pantry with convenient, healthful snacks and foods that you can enjoy once your baby is born. In addition to saving you time and effort, doing this can guarantee that you and your child have access to enough food and nourishment. The following advice will help you prepare your freezer and pantry for life after childbirth:

1. Select shelf-stable, frozen, or canned foods; these include dried fruits, canned fruits, canned vegetables, canned soups, frozen bread, frozen pizza, frozen meat, poultry, and fish, as well as grains, pasta, rice, beans, lentils, nuts, and seeds.

2. Pick meals that are simple to cook, reheat, or prepare, like stir-fry, casserole, pizza, burgers, tortillas, cheese, soup, salad, dressing, eggs, granola, yogurt, cheese, eggs, milk, juice, tea, coffee, crackers, bread, peanut butter, jam, hummus, salsa, and tortillas.

3. Eat a wide variety of nutrient-dense, well-balanced foods from all the food groups, such as grains, fruits, vegetables, dairy products, and healthy fats.

4. Select meals that suit your needs and preferences and are enticing, fulfilling, and versatile. Experiment with a range of flavors, textures, and temperatures, including crunchy, sweet, sour, and hot.

5. Date and label your snacks and foods, keep them in airtight bags or containers, arrange them according to category and

expiration date, and consume them within the suggested amount of time.

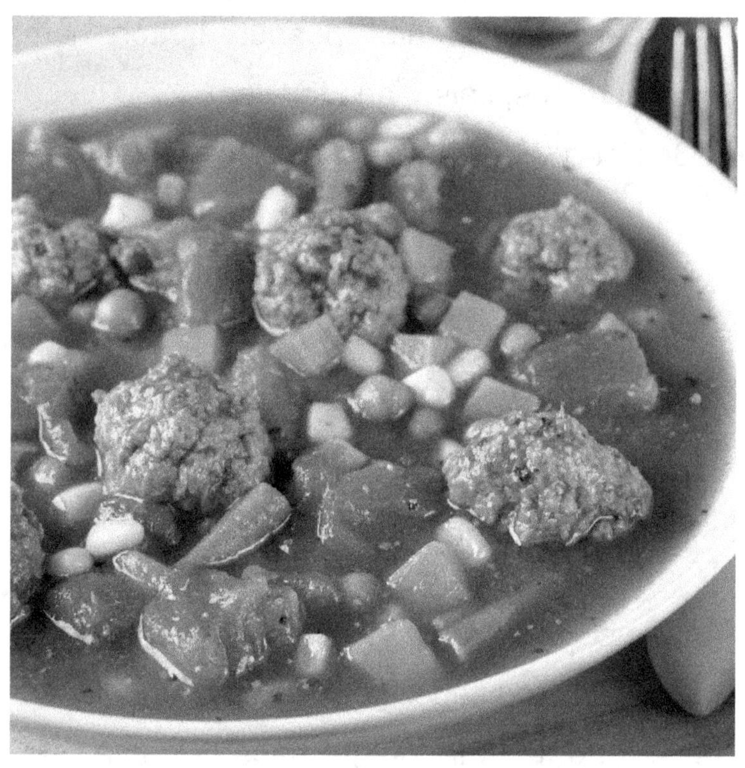

CHAPTER 5

RECIPES FOR OCCASIONS AND CRAVINGS

Being pregnant is a joyful and appreciative time when you are growing and supporting a new life inside of you. Along with enjoying food and life with your loved ones, it's a time for fun and pleasure. It's crucial to eat a healthy, balanced diet for both you and your unborn child, but that doesn't mean you have to deny yourself of treats and cravings. As long as you eat in moderation and with awareness, you are free to indulge in your favorite foods and snacks.

How to Give in to Your Desires and Treats

Cravings and treats are snacks and meals that you like or crave but aren't always wholesome or well-balanced. They frequently have low fiber, vitamin, and mineral content and high sugar, fat, salt, or calorie content. Sweets such as chocolates, pastries, popcorn, chips, ice cream, pizza, burgers, fries, and more may be included. Although cravings and treats don't necessarily pose a health risk, overindulging in them can have negative effects on both your own and your baby's health. Here are some pointers for giving in to cravings and treats:

Recognize your triggers and patterns: Physical elements like hunger, thirst, exhaustion, or hormones can cause certain threats and cravings. Some are brought on by emotional variables like boredom, stress, happiness, or sadness. Certain times of the day, week, or month bring with them greater frequency or intensity of cravings for certain treats. You may better anticipate and control your cravings and treats by becoming aware of your triggers and patterns, which will help you prevent overindulging or bingeing.

Prioritize quality over quantity: Select high-quality, low-quantity foods and snacks when indulging in sweets and cravings. Quality is defined as having a rich, fulfilling, and delectable taste and being prepared with natural, wholesome, and fresh ingredients. The concept of quantity refers to the small, sensible, and appropriate serving sizes of the foods and snacks that are consumed, as well as the moderation of their frequency of consumption. You can indulge in your cravings and treats without endangering your health or the health of your unborn child by prioritizing quality over quantity.

Balance and make up for it: When you give in to temptations and indulgences, make up for it with other meals and pastimes. Incorporating other foods from all the food groups, such as grains, fruits, vegetables, dairy, protein, and healthy fats, into your diet and eating a range of nutrient-dense, well-balanced, and varied foods are examples of maintaining balance. To maintain a healthy weight and lifestyle, compensate by modifying your calorie intake and expenditure and engaging in moderate to frequent exercise. You can avoid or lessen the negative consequences of overindulging, such as weight gain, blood sugar spikes, or nutrient deficiencies, by compensating for and balancing your treats and cravings.

Recipes to Fulfill Cravings and Special Occasions

Cookies with chocolate chips

Soft, chewy, and chocolatey, these cookies are a classic and enticing treat. Additionally, they are simple to store and bake, which can help you avoid or lessen boredom and hunger. They contain chocolate chips, which are high in sugar and antioxidants, butter, which is high in fat and flavor, and flour, which is high in complex and carbs.

Components

- 3/4 cup softened unsalted butter
- 2 cups all-purpose flour
- 1/2 teaspoon baking soda
- 3/4 cup brown sugar

- 1/4 cup granulated sugar
- 1 egg - 1 teaspoon vanilla extract
- One cup of semisweet chocolate chips
- 1/4 teaspoon salt

Guidelines

- Adjust the oven temperature to 350°F and place parchment paper on two baking sheets.
- Using an electric mixer, cream the butter, brown sugar, and granulated sugar in a large bowl until the mixture is light and fluffy. Beat well after adding the egg and vanilla.
- Mix the salt, baking soda, and flour in a medium-sized bowl. When a soft dough forms, gradually combine the dry ingredients with the wet ones and stir. Add the chocolate chips and stir.

- Drop onto the prepared baking sheets by rounded tablespoonfuls, allowing about 2 inches of space between each.
- Bake for ten to twelve minutes, until the centers are set and the edges are golden.
- After allowing the cookies to cool slightly on the baking sheets, move them to a wire rack to finish cooling.
- Savor it with a cup of tea or a glass of milk.

Cheese and Onion Dip

Because it's creamy, cheesy, and oniony, this dip is a great party food. It's also simple to prepare and serve, so you can enjoy your special occasions and wow your family and friends. It has sour cream, which is high in fat and flavor, cream cheese, which is high in calcium and protein, and onion soup mix, which is high in flavor and sodium.

Components

- One package (8 ounces) of softened cream cheese
- One cup of sour cream
- One package (1 ounce) of onion soup mix
- Two tablespoons of freshly chopped parsley
- A variety of chips, crackers, or veggies to dip

Guidelines

- Using an electric mixer, beat the cream cheese in a medium-sized bowl until it becomes smooth. Beat in the onion soup mix and sour cream until thoroughly blended.

- After incorporating the parsley, move the dip into a serving dish.
- Place in the refrigerator until cold and solid, at least one hour.
- Enjoy with vegetables, chips, or crackers.

Brownies

These brownies are fudgy, chocolatey, and moist, making them a rich and decadent treat. Additionally, they are simple to cut and bake, which can help you avoid or lessen boredom and hunger. They contain butter, which is high in fat and flavor, sugar, which is high in calories and sweetness, and cocoa powder, which is rich in antioxidants and flavor.

Components

- 1/2 cup melted unsalted butter
- A cup of powdered sugar and two eggs
- One teaspoon of extract from vanilla

- 1/3 cup of unsweetened cocoa powder
- 1/2 cup of all-purpose flour
- One-fourth teaspoon baking powder
- One-fourth teaspoon salt
- half a cup semisweet chocolate chips

Guidelines

- Grease an 8 x 8-inch baking pan with cooking spray and preheat the oven to 350°F.
- Beat the butter, sugar, eggs, and vanilla together thoroughly in a sizable bowl.
- Sift the flour, baking powder, cocoa powder, and salt in a medium-sized bowl. When a smooth batter forms, gradually add the dry ingredients to the wet ones and stir. Add the chocolate chips and stir.
- Pour the batter into the baking pan, making sure to distribute it evenly.

- A toothpick inserted in the center should come out clean or with a few moist crumbs after baking for 25 to 30 minutes.
- After allowing the brownies to cool fully in the pan, cut them into sixteen squares.
- Savor it with an ice cream scoop or a glass of milk.

Popcorn

This crunchy, salty, and buttery popcorn makes for an easy and satisfying snack. It is also simple to prepare and alter, allowing you to experiment with different flavors and cuisines and diversify your diet. It has butter, which has a lot of fat and flavor, salt, which has a lot of sodium and flavor, and popcorn kernels, which are high in fiber and complex carbohydrates.

Components

- 1/4 cup of kernels for popcorn
- Two tablespoons of melted unsalted butter
- Two tablespoons of vegetable oil
- To taste salt

Guidelines

- Heat the oil in a big pot with a tight-fitting lid over medium-high heat. Cover the pot after adding the popcorn kernels. Shake the pot periodically for three to five minutes or until the popping stops.
- Spoon the popcorn into a sizable bowl and cover with butter. Add a little salt, then toss to coat.
- Savor it with a cup of tea or a glass of water.

Chocolate Avocado Mousse

ingredients

- 1/4 cup cocoa powder
- 2 ripe avocados, pitted and peeled
- One teaspoon vanilla extract,
- one-fourth cup honey or maple syrup,
- a pinch of salt,
- fresh berries for garnish (if desired)

Guidelines

- Place the ripe avocados, cocoa powder, honey (or maple syrup), vanilla extract, and a dash of salt in a food processor or blender.
- Blend, scraping down the sides as necessary, until creamy and smooth.
- Taste and add more honey or maple syrup to adjust sweetness if needed.

- Spoon the mousse made of chocolate and avocado into ramekins or serving dishes.
- To allow the flavors to mingle, refrigerate for a minimum of half an hour before serving.
- If desired, garnish with fresh berries before serving.
- Savor this decadent and healthful dessert on a special day or to sate a chocolate craving!

Caprese Grilled Cheese Sandwich

Ingredients:

- 2 medium tomatoes, thinly sliced
- 4 slices of bread (whole grain or sourdough recommended)
- 4 slices of mozzarella cheese
- Handful of fresh basil leaves
- 2 tablespoons balsamic glaze (optional)

- Olive oil or butter for grilling

Guidelines

- Turn up the heat to medium in a skillet or grill pan.
- To assemble the sandwiches, place two slices of bread together and top with mozzarella cheese, tomato slices, and fresh basil leaves.
- Apply a thin layer of butter or olive oil to the sandwich exteriors.
- Put the sandwiches in the skillet or grill pan and cook for 3–4 minutes on each side, or until they are golden brown and the cheese is melted.
- Drizzle the sandwiches with balsamic glaze, if using, right before serving.
- Present the hot Caprese grilled cheese sandwiches with a side order of soup or salad.

- Satisfy your craving with this gourmet take on a traditional comfort food!

Loaded Sweet Potato Nachos

Ingredients:

- 2 large sweet potatoes, sliced into rounds 1 tablespoon olive oil
- 1 teaspoon chili powder
- 1/2 teaspoon paprika
- 1 teaspoon cumin
- Taste and adjust salt and pepper.
- A single cup of black beans, cooked
- 1/4 cup diced red onion;
- 1/4 cup diced tomatoes;
- 1/4 cup sliced black olives;
- 1 cup shredded cheese (cheddar or Mexican blend);
- Sour cream or Greek yogurt to serve - Fresh cilantro for garnish (optional)

Guideline

- Set the oven's temperature to 400°F, or 200°C. For lining a baking sheet, use parchment paper.
- Evenly coat the sweet potato rounds in a big bowl of olive oil, cumin, paprika, chili powder, salt, and pepper.
- Place the seasoned sweet potato rounds on the baking sheet that has been prepared in a single layer.
- Bake the sweet potatoes for 20 to 25 minutes in a preheated oven, turning them over halfway through, or until they are soft and gently browned.
- Take the baking sheet out of the oven and mix the shredded cheese and black beans with the cooked sweet potato rounds
- Put the baking sheet back in the oven and continue baking for another five to

seven minutes, or until the cheese is bubbling and melted.

- Take the loaded sweet potato nachos out of the oven and garnish them with fresh cilantro, Greek yogurt or sour cream, diced avocado, red onion, and tomatoes.
- Serve right away as a flavorful and filling snack or appetizer for a special occasion or anytime you're in the mood for something substantial and robust!

These recipes, with their delectable flavors and nutritious ingredients, are sure to sate cravings and add even more special memories to any occasion!

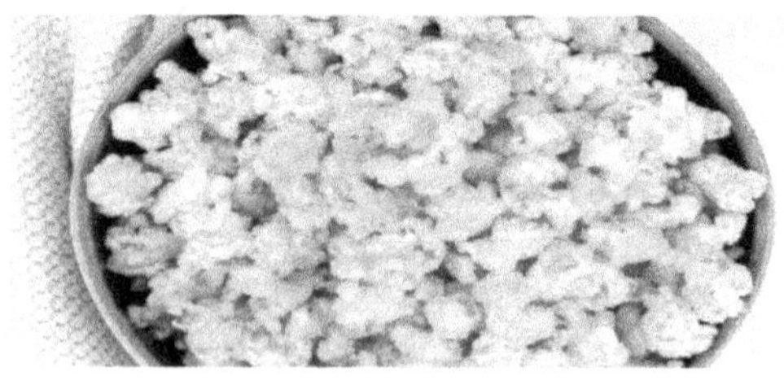

CONCLUSION

As much as I have enjoyed writing this book, I hope you have enjoyed reading it as well.You have reached the end of it. This book was created to give you easy, tasty, and nutritious recipes that you can customize to your preferences and needs to help you eat well and healthily throughout your pregnancy. In this book, we have discussed the following subjects:

- The fundamentals of nutrition and pregnancy, including how to create a diet plan and achieve your dietary objectives
- First-trimester recipes and strategies for managing fatigue, nausea, and food aversions

- Second-trimester recipes: how to satisfy your needs for calories and protein while also promoting your health and the development of your unborn child
- Recipes for special occasions and cravings, along with advice on how to indulge in sweets and cravings mindfully and in moderation - Recipes for the third trimester, including how to deal with heartburn, constipation, swelling, and nesting

You can make sure that you and your infant are getting adequate energy, protein, carbs, fat, vitamins, and minerals by following the suggestions, guidance, and recipes in this book. You can also make sure that you are eating a diverse range of foods that are nourishing, well-balanced, and interesting. You can also celebrate the happiness and thankfulness of being pregnant, as well as the food and the experience.

I wish you all the best for your delivery and postpartum, and I congratulate you on your journey and accomplishment. You should be proud of yourself because you have taken excellent care of both yourself and your child. Recall that food may bring you joy and happiness in addition to providing you with nutrition. So, bon appetit and enjoy both the meal and the occasion!